CW00495579

NURSE
AT THE TRENCHES

Agnes Warner

First Published in 1917 as 'My Beloved Poilus'
by Barnes & Co. Ltd,
St. John, New Brunswick, Canada.

ISBN 1846853672
978-1-84685-367-8

Published in the United Kingdom, April 2005, ISBN 0951565567
Revised Edition published 2006, ISBN 1846853672
by Diggory Press, an imprint of Meadow Books,
Three Rivers, Minions, Liskeard, Cornwall, PL14 5LE
Website: www.diggorypress.com

Printed on acid free paper

These home letters from a Canadian girl, daughter of a retired general of the U.S. Army, giving her trained services, caring for the wounded in France at an Army Ambulance and succoring distress wherever she meets it, were published by her friends without her knowledge, simply and solely to raise money to aid her in her work which began on the 4th of August, 1914. Every dollar received from the sale of the book, less bare cost of printing and express charges, went to the fund.

Preface

WHEN Florence Nightingale began her great work in the hospital wards at Scutari in 1854, she little realised how far-reaching would be the effect of her noble self-sacrificing efforts. Could she today visit the war-stricken countries of Europe she would be astonished at the great developments of the work of caring for the wounded soldiers which she inaugurated so long ago. Her fine example is being emulated today by hundreds of thousands of brave women who are devoting themselves to the wounded, the sick and the dying in countless hospital wards.

All too little is known of what these devoted nurses have done and are doing. Some day the whole story will be given to the world; and the hearts of all will be thrilled by stirring deeds of love and bravery.

In the meantime it is pleasing and comforting to catch fleeting glimpses of a portion of the work as depicted in this sheaf of letters, now issued under the title of 'My Beloved Poilus,' written from the Front by a brave Canadian nurse.

Two outstanding features give special merit to these letters. They were not written for publication, but for an intimate circle of relatives and friends. And because of this they are not artificial, but are free and graceful, with homely touches here and there which add so much to their value.

Amidst the incessant roar of mighty guns; surrounded by the wounded and the dying; shivering at times with cold, and wearied almost to the point of exhaustion, these letters were hurriedly penned. No time had she for finely-turned phrases. Neither were they necessary. The simple statements appeal more to the heart than most eloquent words.

These letters will bring great comfort to many who have loved ones at the Front. They will tell them something of the careful sympathetic treatment the wounded receive. The glimpses given here and there, of the efforts made by surgeons and nurses alike to administer relief, and as far as possible to assuage the suffering of the wounded, should prove most comforting. What efforts are made to cheer the patients, and to brighten their lot, and what personal interest is taken in their welfare, are incidentally revealed in these letters.

For instance, 'The men had a wonderful Christmas Day (1916). They were like a happy lot of children. We decorated the ward with flags, holly and mistletoe, and paper flowers that the men made, and a tree in each ward.'

How these letters bring home to us the terrible tragedy that is going on far across the ocean. And yet mingled with the feeling of sadness is the spirit of inspiration which comes from the thought of those brave men who are offering themselves to maintain the right, and the devoted women who are ministering to their needs. Our heads bow with reverence, and our hearts thrill with pride, when we think of them. But we must do more than think and feel; we must do our part in supporting them and upholding their hands. They have given their all. They can do no more, and dare we do less?

Rev. H. A. Cody. St. John, N. B.,
February 19th, 1917

Introduction

THE writer of these letters, a graduate of McGill College, and the Presbyterian Hospital, New York, left New York in the Spring of 1914 with a patient, for the Continent, finally locating at Divonne-Les-Bains, France, near the Swiss border, where they were on August 1st when war broke out.

She immediately began giving her assistance in 'Red Cross' work, continuing same until the latter part of November, when she returned with her patient to New York, made a hurried visit to her home in St. John and after Christmas returned to again take up the work which these letters describe.

My Beloved Poilus*

Divonne-Les-Bains, France,
August 2, 1914.

Dear Mother

The awful war we have all been dreading is upon us - *France is mobilizing*. At five o'clock yesterday morning the tocsin sounded from the Marie (village hall) and men, women, and children, all flocked to hear the proclamation which the Mayor of the village read. It called upon all of military age - between twenty years and fifty years - to march at once, and inside of twenty-four hours five hundred men had gone, they knew not where. The bravery of these villagers - men and women - is remarkable, and not to be forgotten. No murmuring, no complaining - just, 'Ma Patrie,' tying up the little bundle - so little - and going; none left but old men, women and children.

We have started teaching the women and girls to make bandages, sponges, etc., for the hospital which will be needed here.

* Editor's note: Poilus was an affectionate term for the unshaven fighting men in the trenches.

Divonne-Les-Bains, France
August 23, 1914.

Your letter came yesterday - twenty days on the way - but I was fortunate to get it at all; so many of these poor people, whose nearest and dearest have gone to fight for their country, have had no word from them since they marched away, and they do not know where they are.

From this little village 500 men left the first day of mobilization; there is not a family who has not some one gone, and from some both fathers and sons have gone, as the age limit is from twenty to fifty years.

I am filled with admiration and respect for these people. The courage of both the men and women is remarkable. There is no hesitation, and no grumbling, and everyone tries to do whatever he or she can to help the cause.

I do not know if I told you, in my last letter, of the poor lady who walked all night through the dark and storm to see her son who was leaving the next morning. All the horses and motors had been taken by the Government for the army, so she started at eleven o'clock at night, all by herself, and got here about five in the morning - her son left at seven, so she had two hours with him. While there are such mothers in France she cannot fall. There are many such stories I might tell you, but I have not the time.

The 'Red Cross' has started a branch hospital here, and I have been helping them to get it in order. It is just about ready now, and we may get soldiers any day.

I have classes every morning and find many of the women very quick to learn the rudiments of nursing.

Everyone in the place is making supplies and our sitting room is a sort of depot where they come for work.

If my patient is as well in October as she is now I am going to stay and give my services to the 'Red Cross.' If I have to go home with her I will come back - I would be a coward and deserter if I did not do all I could for these poor brave people.

October 25, 1914.

Another Sunday - but this is cold and rainy - the days slip by so quickly I cannot keep track of them. We have only two soldiers left at the hospital - they tell us every day that others are coming. The country all about is perfectly beautiful with the autumn coloring.

We do not see any of the horrors of the war here. If it were not for the tales that come to us from outside, and for the poor broken men who come back, we would not know it was going on. There are very enthusiastic accounts of the Canadians in all the English papers.

Paris, about February 15, 1915.

Back safely in Paris after taking my patient to New York and a short visit home, which now seems like a dream.

I have been spending a lot of time at the American Ambulance this week, but have not gone out to stay as yet, as I still have to see some other small hospitals and had to go to the Clearing House to make arrangements for sending supplies, which I brought from home and New York, to different places.

I have seen quite a number of operations, and as X-ray pictures are taken of all the cases there is no time wasted in hunting for a bullet; they get the bullet out in about two minutes. They are using Dr. Criles' anæsthetic - nitrous oxide gas and oxygen - it has no bad effects whatever.

The patients come out of it at once as soon as the mask is taken off, and there is no nausea or illness at all; and most of them go off laughing, for they cannot believe that it is all over - they feel so well; but oh, mother, it is awful to see the sad things that have happened.

In some cases there are only pieces of men left. One young chap, twenty-one years old, has lost both legs. At first he did not want to live, but now he is beginning to take an interest in things and is being fitted for wooden legs.

The dental department have done wonderful work. They build up the frame work of the face and jaws and then the surgeons finish the work by making new noses and lips and eyelids.

I thought I had seen a good many wonderful things, but I did not believe it possible to make anything human out of some of the pieces of faces that were left, and in some of the cases they even get rid of the scars. Photos are taken when they first come in, and then in the various stages of recovery.

One of the worst cases I saw the last day I was out. He has to have one more operation to fill in a small hole in one side of his nose and then he will be all right.

Last Sunday one of the men in Miss B's ward was given the medal for distinguished service. He had saved his officer's life - went right out before the guns and carried him in on his back. He was struck himself just before he got to his own lines and one leg almost torn off.

When they brought him to the American Ambulance, all the doctors, except Dr. B, said his leg would have to come off at once - he refused to do it and saved the leg for the man. It will be stiff, of course, as the knee joint is gone entirely; but will be better than a wooden leg, and the poor man is so pleased.

I must tell you about the wonderful dog that is at the American Ambulance; perhaps you have read about him in some of the papers. His master came from Algeria, and of course did not expect to take his dog with him, but when the ship left the wharf the dog jumped into the sea and swam after it, so they put off a boat and hauled him on board, and he has been with his master all through the war.

He was in the trenches with him, and one day a German shell burst in the trench and killed all of his companions and buried this man in the mud and dirt as well as injuring him terribly. Strange to say the dog was not hurt at all, and the first thing the man remembered was the dog digging the mud off his face. As soon as he realized his master was alive he ran off for help, and when they were brought into the Ambulance together there were not many dry eyes about.

After he was sure his master was being taken care of he consented to go and be fed, and now he is having the time of his life. He is the most important person in the place. He has a beautiful new collar and medal, lives in the diet kitchen, and is taken out to walk by the nurses, and best of all is allowed to see his master every day.

I will send a photo of him to you. His master has lost one leg, the other is terribly crushed, and one hand also, but Doctor B. thinks he can save them.

I think I shall go back to Divonne-Les-Bains - they are urging me so strongly and there seems to be more need there.

February 19, 1915.

Back again in Divonne-Les-Bains. It seems as if I had never been away - I have fallen into the old work so easily. I left Paris Sunday night about eight o'clock and arrived here at two the next day, and had a warm welcome from everybody. One poor man died of tetanus before I got back. I have nine on my floor. I have thirteen patients, nine in bed all the time, and the others up part of the day. One of the women of the village helps me in the morning, two others help with the cleaning up and serving meals; everything has to be carried up three flights of stairs, so you can imagine the work.

I have a very comfortable room at the hotel, go to the Ambulance at seven in the morning and generally get back at nine or half past. I do not know how long I shall be here - until this lot get well or more come.

One of the patients is a chef, and was acting as cook for the regiment when a shell landed in his soup pot; he was not wounded, but his heart was knocked out of place by the shock and his back was twisted when he fell.

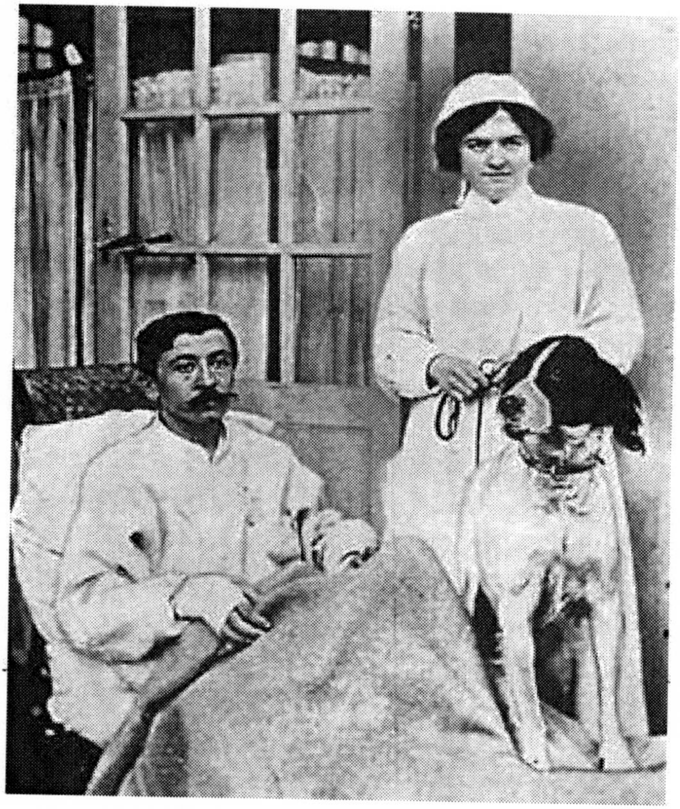

The dog who saved his master's life.

February 28, 1915.

The poor man who was so very ill died on the morning of the twenty-third after three weeks of intense suffering - I stayed that night with him. The others are all out of danger with the exception of two who cannot get well - one is paralyzed and the other has tuberculosis.

I went to the village for the first time yesterday and was quite touched by the welcome I received at every little shop and house. The people seemed genuinely glad to have me back. They cannot seem to get over the fact that I have crossed the ocean twice and come back to them. To them the ocean is a thing of terror, especially since the war broke out.

Doctor R has a great many sick people in the country about here to take care of in addition to the soldiers. In one house they had nothing to eat but potatoes, but he is a good deal like our dear old doctor, and feeds and clothes and takes care of them himself.

March 5, 1915.

I can scarcely believe that it is nearly three weeks since I left Paris. I have been so busy, that the days fly by. Some of the men are leaving tomorrow, and most of the others are getting along very well.

Mr. E is indeed kind. He has just sent an order to the village people, who make beautiful lace and embroidery, for $500.00 worth of work. They are so happy about it, for it means food for many of them. One poor woman, who has lost her husband in the war and has a child to take care of, can earn only eighteen francs a month, that is $3.60, and that is all she has to live on.

March 7, 1915.

One of the American doctors from the American Ambulance came to see me yesterday. He was very much interested in what he saw and is coming back in ten days. We have had one or two beautiful days, the pussy-willows are beginning to come out, and primroses everywhere.

Dr. S said that the man who owned the wonderful dog that is at the American Ambulance is really getting well, and they managed to save one leg and the crushed hand.

In Dr. B's service he did not do a single amputation during the months of January and February - a very wonderful record.

Dr. S seems to think there is no hope of my poor paralyzed man getting better, he may live for twenty years but can never walk. I am giving him English lessons every day. He is very quick at learning; it helps pass the time. Poor man, he has already been in bed six months.

March 21, 1915.

This has been the most lovely Spring day. The violets are blooming in the fields, they are smaller than ours but very fragrant; the yellow primroses are beautiful and grow everywhere. There is still lots of snow on the mountains but none in the valley. If it were not for the soldiers who are here we could scarcely believe that terrible fighting is going on so near us.

A lot of our men went off last week, some of them scarcely able to hobble, poor things, but all the hospitals are being cleared out to make room for the freshly wounded. We are expecting a new lot every day, and have prepared ten extra beds.

I will have some letters this week to send to the 'Red Cross' and 'The De Monts' Chapter, I. O. D. E., thanking them for the things they sent back by me; they have been so much appreciated, done so much good and relieved so much distress. I gave some to Mademoiselle de C who sent them to a small hospital in Normandy near their chateau, some to the hospital here, and some to a small hospital not far from here where they are very poor; the doctor who is in charge there nearly wept when he knew the things were for him.

March 26, 1915.

Another beautiful day and the air is soft and balmy as a day in June. The woods and fields are full of spring flowers, there are big soft gray pussies on all the willow trees and the other trees are beginning to show a faint tinge of green. It is certainly a lovely place.

You probably felt much relieved that I was not in Paris at the time of the last air raid when the bombs were dropped. One fell so near the Ambulance at Neuilly that one of the doctors was knocked out of bed by the shock.

I had my paralyzed man out on the balcony today, it is the first time in six months that he has been out. One of the men here, who has lost the use of both hands, told me today that he had six brothers in the army; two have been killed, two wounded and two are still at the front. He was a coachman in a private family, has lost a thumb of one hand and on the other has only the thumb and one finger left. Fortunately his employer is a good man and will take care of him; but think of the poor man - horses are his chief joy, and he will never be able to drive again.

April 2, 1915.

Easter Sunday and still raining. We had a splendid service from Mr. - and a Communion service after. The service is more like the Presbyterian than any other. We have four new soldiers but the large convoy has not yet arrived. There has been awful fighting in Alsace lately, so the wounded must come soon.

Today we had a specially good dinner for the men. Madam B gave them cigars and Easter eggs, and after dinner they sang some of their songs, then gave us three cheers. They are a fine lot of men and so grateful for every thing we do for them.

The story of the dog has gone through the whole country, but it is nice to know that it is really true, and to have seen the dog. Dr. B was able to save the other leg of the dog's master, and after another operation he thinks he will have the use of his hand.

April 10, 1915.

We had a severe snow storm today and yesterday also, and in between the snow storms it poured rain; all the lovely spring weather has disappeared.

Wednesday night they announced the arrival of a train of wounded, for the next morning at half-past five, but did not tell us how many to expect. We all went to the Ambulance at half-past five and got everything ready for dressing and beds prepared for thirty. At seven thirteen arrived - all convalescents, and no dressings at all to do. The last time forty came, and all in a dreadful state of infection, so we never know what to expect.

I am not sorry I came back to Divonne for I feel that I have been able to help more here than in Paris; there they have many to help and here very few.

I am sending you a photo of three of my patients - Chasseurs d' Alpine or 'Blue Devils' as the Germans call them - they are the ones who have done such wonderful work in Alsace.

April 19, 1915.

I have had quite a busy week, for my men have been coming and going. The paralyzed man has been sent to Bourg, the two Chasseurs d' Alpine have gone and I have six new ones - this lot is ill, not wounded. There are three officers among them - one is a cousin of Madam B, the French lady who helped establish this Ambulance. Her husband came on Thursday; he has eight days leave. He is very interesting, for he has been all up through the north of France. He is adjutant to one of the generals and travels from eighty to one hundred miles a day in a motor, carrying despatches. There is a French aviator here, but he has not got his machine, so I am afraid there is no hope for me.

April 25, 1915.

They took down all the stoves in the Ambulance last week, and the day after it snowed; we had to put some of the men to bed to keep them warm. We have been very busy all week, new patients coming every day till now we have forty. Most of them are not wounded. Poor fellows, they are utterly done out; some have pneumonia, others rheumatism, one paralyzed and all sorts of other things.

This is a wonderful place for them to come to and most of them get well very quickly. They are talking of increasing the number of beds in the hospital and of making it a regular military one. In that case they will send a military doctor here and the whole thing will be re-organized. They want me to promise to take charge of it, but I do not think it would be a wise thing, there is so much red tape and so many things about the military organization I do not understand, that I am afraid I would get into hot water at once.

I am sending you a circular of Mademoiselle de Canomonts' lace school. They do lovely work and need all the help and orders that they can get. They will be glad to execute orders by mail for anyone writing them to Divonne-Les-Bains, France.

May 2, 1915.

I have never seen anything as lovely as the country is now, it is like one great garden; how I wish you could be here. I have had a busy day, as one of my patients had to be operated on. Doctor R took a piece of shrapnel out of his arm, and two others have been pretty ill; four leave tomorrow, so the general clearing up will begin again.

My poor old lady who had a stroke of paralysis died yesterday. I have been helping take care of her. The only son is at the front. So many old people are dying this year; when they get ill they don't seem to have any power of resistance; poor things, they have endured so much they cannot stand any more.

There is a poor little woman here who comes from Dinant, that was destroyed by the Germans in the early part of the war. She has lost all trace of her father and mother; her husband and brother have both been killed and their property utterly destroyed. Mr. B, the pastor of the Protestant Church, has not been able to find his mother, who disappeared last August. Every day we hear of something new.

The papers are full of accounts of the gallant fighting of the Canadians, but the losses have been very heavy.

May 9, 1915.

It is just a year today since I sailed from New York, starting on our trip with Mrs. E.. Little did we think of the horrors that have happened since.

Seven more men went off last night, so we have only twenty left. I have ten on my floor, but only four in bed; the others are able to be out all day. Charrel, one of my patients who just left, was one of six brothers, all of whom went off the first days of the war; three have been killed, the other three wounded.

I am going to Lyons on Thursday for a few days to visit some of the hospitals.

The French papers are full of the heroism of the Canadian troops; they have done wonderful work at Ypres, but at what a terrible cost.

I feel so proud every time I see the dressing gowns the DeMonts Chapter sent me - they are the nicest we have.

May 18, 1915.

I left here Thursday at noon with Madam B who went to Paris. Before I left I telegraphed to Madam M , the wife of the soldier who was here such a long time, asking her to get me a room, but when I arrived I found the whole family at the station to meet me and they insisted on my going home to stay with them. They are very simple people, but so kind and hospitable. I think it is quite an event having a stranger stay with them. We ate in the kitchen, and the whole family seemed to sleep in a cupboard opening off of it.

I saw a lot of hospitals and was rather favorably impressed with them. At the Hotel Dieu, they had received seven hundred patients within twenty-four hours. I think the saddest part was the eye ward, there were so many who would never see again and some of them so young. There were some with both legs gone and others both feet, and many with one arm or leg missing.

The boats on the river that were fitted up as hospitals were very interesting, but I fancy would be very hot in the summer and the mosquitoes would be terrible.

Saturday I spent the day with Mademoiselle R, who had been staying at the Hotel at Divonne for a time.

The R's are a wealthy family who have lived in Lyons for generations. Mademoiselle was able to take me to a good many of the hospitals, as they have done a good deal for them. We visited them in the morning, which was much more interesting, as we saw the work going on.

At two of the hospitals wounded were arriving when we left there, so we saw the whole thing. I also saw the dressing being done in one of the large military hospitals. In the afternoon we went to a 'Red Cross' hospital, where she worked in the lingerie; there are fifty beds and the patients are taken care of by the sisters. They seemed to be very cheerful and well looked after.

Sunday morning I got up at 3.30 and took a train at 4.30 for Romans where Mrs. C is working in a military hospital. At eight I arrived at Tourons and had to walk from there to a small village called Tain, where I got a tramway to Romans. I arrived at eleven, had my lunch on the sidewalk before a cafe - a most excellent meal for fifty cents.

I found Mrs. C at the convent, where she is staying; fortunately she had the afternoon off. She has charge of the dressings and all of the infected operations. At the hospital where she is they have forty wounded Germans; they seem very contented and glad to be there. Mrs. C says it is dreadful to do their dressings, for they have no self-control at all; they have a certain dogged courage that makes them fight as they do, in the face of certain death, but when they are wounded they cannot stand the pain. The French, on the contrary, seldom say a word; they will let one do anything, and if the pain is very bad they moan occasionally or say a swear word, but I have never seen one who lost control of himself and screamed.

I had dinner with Mrs. C at the convent, and at 7.15 took the train for Valence where I changed and waited two hours for the train to Lyons, but there was so much going on at the station that the time did not seem long - troops coming and going all the time and a hospital train with three hundred wounded arrived.

Monday morning I left for Divonne and arrived back very tired but well satisfied with my trip. I found two new patients, one with a leg as big as an elephant and the other out of his head. I have twelve now on my floor.

Just think! Lily of the valley grows wild here, and you can get a bushel in a morning; the whole place is sweet with the perfume

May 28, 1915

We got twelve more patients Wednesday - six left. I still have fifteen; this lot were all ill. One man is quite a character. The doctor put him on milk diet the first day - but he did not approve, so he went to the village and bought a loaf of bread and some ham.

Between the florist of the village and the wife of one of the soldiers I am kept well supplied with roses. I wish I could share my riches with you.

I am anxiously waiting to hear of the safe arrival of the Twenty-fourth; as we have heard nothing, they must be all right. It is hard to have them go but I cannot understand the attitude of those who will not go or who object to their men and boys going. You are just beginning to feel now what they have been suffering here since August last.

Madam L.H. was called back to Verdun today; she was supposed to have three weeks' holidays, but has only been away ten days. She is not fit to go back but there is no help for it.

There was great excitement here when Italy finally declared war. It is awful to think of the brutes throwing bombs on Venice. I do hope they will not do any harm there.

I must say goodnight, for I am tired. I am up at half-past five every morning and seldom get off duty before nine at night.

June 20, 1915

Yesterday we got five patients - the four worst were consigned to me. One poor chap was shot through the body and the spine was injured; they do not know just what the extent of the injury is, but he is completely paralyzed from the waist down. Fortunately he is very small, so it is not difficult to take care of him; he is the most cheerful soul, and says he has much to be thankful for as he has never suffered at all.

When he was shot he simply had the sensation of his legs disappearing. When he fell he said to a comrade, 'Both my legs have gone,' but he had no pain at all. His comrade assured him that he had not lost his legs, but he said he could not believe it until he got to the hospital. He has received the Médaille Militaire for bravery, and his comrades said he certainly deserved it. He is so glad to get here, where it is real country and quiet. We put him on a chaise longue on the balcony today and he has been out of doors all day long.

It is after ten o'clock, but I am still at the Ambulance. We are waiting for a train that is bringing us fifteen wounded directly from Alsace. Poor souls, they will be glad to get here, for they have been a long time on the way.

No letters this week; regulations are very strict again, and they are holding up all mail for eight or ten days.

June 22, 1915.

I had to stop my letter as the men arrived. We got eighteen instead of fifteen. Such a tired dirty lot they were; they came straight from the battlefield, and had only had one dressing done since they were wounded. Some of them came on stretchers, others were able to walk, as they were wounded in the arms and head.

I drew two from this lot, which brings my number up to seventeen again. One of mine has both bones broken in his leg and the other is wounded in the left side and shoulder. One poor chap had been a prisoner in one of the trenches for four days and they were unable to get any food all that time; most of them have slept ever since they arrived, they were so exhausted.

Today a military doctor came from Besaucon to show us about some special electrical treatment. They are going to increase the beds by fifty to begin with, and later may make it three hundred.

The news is not good today, the Russians seem to be retreating all the time and the losses in the north are terrible.

There seems to be no doubt in the minds of many people that the war will last another year at least; it seems too terrible.

June 27, 1915.

I did not get my letter off today as there was so much to do. We have had inspection all week. They have finally decided to enlarge the hospital very much and make it a semi-military institution of four hundred beds. We are to turn the large dining room into a ward with fifty beds, and the large part of the hotel will hold three hundred more. They want me to take charge. Dr. R will be chief with two assistants.

There will be forty men nurses - convalescent soldiers - and I do not know how many more women nurses. I am very glad it has been so decided, for it is a great pity this place has not been of more use. Our last lot of men are getting on very well now; but we have had a hard week, for some of them were very ill. The doctor was very much afraid one man would lose his arm, but he has managed to save it.

I have grown to be a sort of official shotsnapper for the Ambulance and village. It is really very interesting and my camera is very good.

Did I send you the snaps of the Bayin baby? She is only nine months old and runs around like a rabbit - is as pretty as a picture. I am so sleepy I can hardly see, so goodnight.

July 4, 1915.

I was glad to get your letter this week; three weeks on the way is a long time to wait.

I have such mixed feelings when I hear that the troops have left St. John. My heart aches for those left behind, but I am so glad to know they are on the way, for they are needed badly and they will get a royal welcome, for Canadians have proved their worth.

When they were in barracks and had nothing to do but drill they were not always angels; but when there was real work to be done their equal was not to be found. The French papers were full of the stories of their bravery. There were some officers who said that while others were splendid fighters the Canadians were marvelous.

It must have been terribly hard for Mrs. to let S go. I wish you would ask her for his address. I will try and get in touch with him and if he should be ill or wounded tell her I will go to him if I have to walk to get there. Get D's address also, so I can look after him. When I hear of them all being over here a wave of homesickness comes over me and I feel that I must go and join them.

There is much to be done on this side now, for the fighting in Alsace has been terrible. The last lot of soldiers that came were Chasseurs d' Alpine, and out of one thousand two hundred who went off only five hundred came back, and the greater number of them wounded.

Fifteen young men from this village have been missing since the terrible battle of three weeks ago, the deaths of a half a dozen have been confirmed but of the others nothing is known.

I am afraid there is no chance of the war finishing before the winter is over.

I wish somebody would organize a 'French Day' or 'Divonne Day' and collect pennies for me; we will need so many things before the winter is over. The general who came the other day said to make the money we have go to the furthest possible point, and then make debts - the soldiers must be taken care of.

July 11, 1915.

We have had arrivals and departures all week. The days are not half long enough to do all that is necessary. My four men who came for electrical treatment are getting on wonderfully well, the big one who was paralyzed and who could not move hand or foot when he came, is now walking without crutches, and feeds himself.

The poor little chasseur who was shot through the body is really better. He is beginning to walk - with a great deal of help, of course. He can make the movements of walking and can put both legs straight out in front of him, and the doctor says there is great hope of a permanent cure. Poor little man, he deserves to get well, for I have never seen such courage and patience. We begin tomorrow to prepare the big dining room for fifty new patients, so we shall have a busy week. I am to have charge of the big ward and keep my floor as well. I will have two military men nurses and some more people from the village to help.

July 17, 1915.

We have had a most terrific rain for the last two days - the people are getting anxious on account of the grain.

There was no celebration in the village on the fourteenth as is usual, but at the Ambulance we had a little feast in honor of the men who were at Metezeral. We have four from the Seventh Chasseurs, whose regiment was decorated for unusual bravery.

My paralyzed man stood up alone last Sunday for the first time and now he walks, pushing a chair before him like a baby. He is the happiest thing you can imagine; for seven months he has had no hope of ever walking again.

Seven left last week and six more go on Monday, so we shall probably get a train load before long.

I have got a small English boy to help me in the mornings. He has been at school in Switzerland and the whole will be entirely cured. Daillet wrote to his mother and told her that he could stand alone and was beginning to walk, but she did not believe it; she thought that he was just trying to cheer her up, so he asked me to take a photo of him standing up so that he could send it to her. He was the proudest, happiest thing you can imagine when he sent it off. Then his aunt came to see him, so the poor mother is finally convinced that it is true, and is coming to see him as soon as the haying is done, but she has to work in the fields now and cannot get away.

It is wonderful the work that the women do here. There are only two old horses left in the whole village, so the women harness themselves into the rakes and waggons and pull them in place of the horses - and they so seldom complain of the hard work. I asked one woman if she did not find it very hard, and she said at first it came very difficult but she got used to it and it was nice to be able to do their part.

We got twenty men from Alsace on Friday - some of them badly wounded. They did not arrive till half-past eleven at night, and it was three in the morning before we got the dressings done and got them to bed. It is the second time that some of them have been wounded. They are all Chasseurs d'Alpines - they are a splendid type. Some of them had both legs and both arms wounded. Yesterday we were rather anxious about several of them, but today they are better. They generally sleep about three days after they arrive, they are so done out.

Mrs. H has had to leave to care for a typhoid patient, so my hands are very full. My English boy is getting trained rapidly; he is only seventeen and not very strong, too young to go to the war but very keen to do something to help.

Do not worry about me, I am as well as possible and as strong as a horse, but as my day begins at half-past five in the morning and ends at half-past nine at night I fall asleep over my letters.

Thanks for the clippings; I would not have known B. if the name had not been there. I do not dare to think of his coming, and yet I would not be proud of him if he did not want to come. I shall try and get up to the north later so as to be nearer him when he comes.

Goodnight, mother; these are sad times, but we must not lose courage. I wish I could see you tonight.

August 1, 1915.

To say that I was delighted will not express my feelings when I got the letter from the Loyalist Chapter, I. O. D. E., enclosing cheque. It was awful good of them to help us here, for I realize the demands for help on every side and it is only natural that they should send to the Canadians first. But O! it is so badly needed and will so do much good here. I had been racking my brain trying to think of a way to scratch up a few pennies, and then this delightful surprise came.

This hospital is called the 'Paradise of the Seventh Region,' for it is so very far ahead of most of the French military hospitals. But while there is a good deal of luxury on one side, such as pleasant airy rooms, comfortable beds, good food and air, on the other hand there is a great lack of what we consider necessities. The first thing I did when I got the letter with the money was to order a foot tub for each floor, slippers for the patients when they are in the house, scissors for the pharmacy and for each floor, and various other small things that I have been longing for and that will save many steps.

Now that the capacity of the hospital has been increased by fifty beds, it is more difficult than ever to get money from the general fund for things of that kind; it really has to be kept for food and heating. We also need instruments and basins, etc., for a table for dressings in the new ward, as we have absolutely nothing.

Then it is so nice to have a fund that we can draw on in case of need. Sometimes the men are terribly poor and cannot afford to get anything for themselves when they leave. Sometimes a ticket for a wife or daughter to come to see them and cheer them up. It is the second time some of these men have been wounded and they have not seen their families for a year.

It is just a year today (August 1st) since mobilization began. At five o'clock in the morning the tocsin sounded and all the village gathered at the Town Hall to read the notice of mobilization. There were many sad and anxious hearts then but many more now, for there is not à family who has not lost someone who is near and dear to them - and still it goes on. I wonder when the end will come.

My prize patient, Daillet, walks down stairs by himself now by holding on to the railing like a child. We are all proud of him. The doctor who sent him here from Besaucon came in the other day to see how he was getting on and he could not believe it when he saw him.

I am almost asleep so I must stop. I made a mistake this morning, got up at half-past four instead of half-past five.

August 15, 1915.

In the face of all the terrible things which are happening one must not worry over little things. I have got to the stage now when I feel as if one should never complain or worry if they have a roof over their heads and enough to eat, and that all one's efforts should be given to helping others.

I feel perfectly overwhelmed with the letters that ought to be written, but cannot find time to do them. I have been up all night and a couple of days. We got thirty new patients last night. They arrived at 3 A. M. and it was half past five before we got them to bed. I did not get any of this lot, as my rooms were full. There were not so many wounded, more sick, rheumatism, bronchitis, etc. One poor man said it was like going directly from hell to heaven; it was the first time he had slept in a bed for a year. Some of them have been wounded for the second time. It is nearly eleven and I must be up early, so goodnight.

August 21, 1915.

Your letter has been long delayed, as they are very strict and holding up the mails again.

We heard this morning that there are French troops guarding the border at Crassier, just half a mile from here. We hear all the Swiss border is to be protected by barbed wire. I do not know what it all means unless it is on account of spies.

We got fifteen more patients last week, one yesterday and one today, but as several went away we have still the same number - eighty-four.

We have had a very busy morning. An inspector arrived just as we were ready to operate, and between the two I did not know whether I was on my head or my heels. Thirty of our men will go off on Monday and we will probably get a train full later in the week.

We have a phonograph with a rasping voice that plays from morning to night. The soldiers love it; the poor things are so used to noise that they don't seem happy without it, but sometimes I feel as if I could scream.

One of the men got a telegram saying his mother was dying; the doctor gave him forty-eight hours leave - all he could possibly do - so he went home and has just got back; could not stay for the funeral, but was so thankful to have been able to see her. If he had been at the front that would not have been possible - only another sad consequence of the war. Another soldier received the news of the death of his little girl.

Miss Todd took me out in her motor the other day. We had a beautiful run over the mountains; the view was magnificent. We took one of the soldiers with us and he enjoyed himself immensely; it was the first time he had ever been in one.

Sunday, August 29, 1915.

It is pouring rain, it is sad to say, as the soldiers are having a little celebration. A band came from Nejon and the Count de Divonne made a speech, two of the men received their Croix de Guerre, the doctor made such a nice little speech to each of them. It was very touching to see the groups of men, some with arms in slings and others with legs and heads bandaged, and some who could not stand at all, still others were in their beds. The decorations were given in the Grand Salle.

I am not sure if all your letters reach me or not, sometimes I get two in a week and then again none for three weeks.

Thirty-three men go off tomorrow, some of them cured and back to the front, some who will never be better, and some to go home on convalescence.

Today the florist in the village sent a clothes basket full of roses to the Ambulance for the fete. I thought of you and wished you could have some.

September 5, 1915.

Thanks for the money you sent from a friend in your last letter. I will use it wisely and make it go as far as possible. There will be more suffering this winter than there was last, but they are so brave, these people, they seldom complain of anything.

There is a little woman here whose husband was killed. She makes twenty cents a day selling papers and gets ten cents a day pension. She has three children, the eldest a girl of twelve. I got her a good pair of boots the other day and warm underclothes for the other children. She was so grateful.

Don't worry about me. My expenses are very small, I have not bought any clothes and do not need any this winter.

Today they had a big concert in the hotel, the proceeds go to the Ambulance.

We have had an awful week of rain and cold, but hope for a little more sunshine to thaw us out.

Our good doctor is going to be married next month. I am so glad, for he lives all alone and needs some one to look after him.

I shall have to go to bed to get warm. There is no heat in this house and when it rains it is like an ice box.

September 11, 1915.

I expect to leave here in two weeks to go to an Ambulance at the front. It is somewhere in the north in Belgium. I think Dr. R is sorry to have me leave, but it will be a much larger field and the kind of a place where there will be much to do. They have all been so nice to me here about helping me get my papers ready to send to the Minister of War, so I do not think there will be any difficulty of my getting through. I go to Paris first, then to Dunkirk, where Mrs. T will meet me, after that my destination is uncertain.

Do not worry if you do not hear from me regularly, for it may be difficult to get mail through. I will write as usual.

I cannot tell you how glad I am to be able to go to the front, for it means a chance to do good work and I shall be so glad to be in the north when B. comes over and nearer the Canadian boys. Even if I cannot see them I shall not feel so far away.

One of my men today got word that his baby, seven months old, had just died and the little girl of two is very ill. He expected to go next week and has been counting the days till he could see them. He has never seen the baby as it was born after the war began - another one of the sad things of this awful war.

Goodnight; I am so glad of the chance of active service.

September 18, 1915.

It was awfully good of Miss W to send the money to me, it is so much needed here. I expect to get off Monday or Tuesday of next week.

September 19, 1915.

My orders came today, and I leave on Tuesday for Paris and on Friday for Dunkirk. I am up to my eyes in work, for there is so much to be done before leaving and new people to break in. Three military nurses arrived yesterday, but it is rather difficult to manage for they know nothing at all about taking care of sick people. They have all been at the front, and wounded too badly to return and sent into an auxiliary service. One is a priest, one a hair dresser and the third a horse dealer; however, they are nice men and are willing to learn, which is a great thing in their favor.

If they are able to raise any money for me I will see that it is wisely spent. There is great need everywhere, and I am proud of the people of St. John, they have done so much.

There is a poor woman who lives in a little village near here. She had two sons - one has been killed in the war, the other a helpless cripple for eighteen years and is not able to move out of his chair. He makes baskets sometimes, but now there is no one to buy the baskets. The mother goes out by the day but can earn so little. I gave him five francs, one of the De Monts dressing gowns and some warm underclothes. He was so grateful, poor boy, and says he will not feel the cold now. His mother is away nearly all day and he sits by the window all alone and depends upon the neighbours coming in to help him from time to time; he is always cheerful and never complains.

The Ws have such a hard time - they get so little of their income since the war began. It has gradually gone down from $3,000.00 per year to $500.00; four of them to live on that amount. So many people are in just the same condition, there is no end to the misery.

I do not know whether it is the French or the English army we are to follow at my new post.

Paris, September 23, 1915.

I am off tomorrow at 7.30 A. M., to Boulogne, then Calais and reach Dunkirk at 9.30 P. M. I have had two very strenuous days and will be glad to rest in the train tomorrow. It took such a time to get my papers in order. The thermometer for the last two days has been about 100.

Mobile NO. 1, France, 1915.

I am really not in France but Belgium. I cannot tell you just where, but it is within ten miles of the firing line, and not far from the place where so many of our boys from home have been sent. I thought when I came here that it would be entirely English, as the lady who gave the hospital is an American married to an Englishman. The English are not far away but they are taken to their own hospitals.

We belong to a little wedge of the French that is in between the English and Belgians. It is a regular field hospital and is composed of a great many portable huts or sheds; some are fitted up as wards, another the operating room, another the pharmacy, another supply room, laundry, nurses' quarters, doctors' quarters, etc. It is a little colony set down in the fields and the streets are wooden sidewalks.

The first night I arrived I did not sleep, for the guns roared all night long, and we could see the flashes from the shells quite plainly; the whole sky was aglow. The French and English guns sounded like a continuous roar of thunder; but when the shells from the German guns landed on this side we could feel a distinct shock, and everything in our little shanty rattled.

Yesterday I saw my first battle in the air between German and French aeroplanes. We could scarcely see the machines, they were so high up in the air, but we could see the flashes from their guns quite distinctly and hear the explosion of the shells. Today a whole fleet of aeroplanes passed over our heads; it was a wonderful sight.

There are about one hundred and fifty beds in all here.

I have been inspected by doctors, captains, generals, and all kinds of people till I am weary. I hope they are satisfied at last, but I cannot go off the hospital grounds until I have two different kinds of passes given to me - one is a permission to go on the roads about here and the other is good as far as Dunkirk.

We have a man in our ward who had a piece of shrapnel the size of an egg in his abdomen; they had to take out about half a yard of intestines, which had been torn to pieces. He was also shot through the shoulder, in the arm and leg. As we got him within two hours after he was wounded there was no infection, and having a clever surgeon he is getting along famously. Another poor chap has lost his right arm and shot through the liver as well as being cut up by piece of shrapnel - he is getting well also. Two have died, and it is a blessing; for to live in darkness the rest of one's life is worse than death. The Germans are using a new kind of gas, bomb that blinds the men.

It is pouring rain tonight and cheerless enough here, but I can only think of the poor men in the trenches.

I got a joyful surprise today - a letter from Mr. Bell enclosing post office order from Mr. Calhoun, of Philadelphia. Nothing gives me so much pleasure as to help these poor people.

It is beginning to get cold. I shall get bed socks for the men, for they have not enough hot water bags to go round and all suffer from cold feet.

I passed Colonel MacLaren's hospital in the train - it is very impressive to see the rows and rows of white tents. I also saw some Canadian nurses in the distance, and did so want to get out and speak to them. I must go to bed now to get warm. As long as one keeps going the cold is not so apparent but when one sits still it is not pleasant.

There are four English, three American and three French nurses here.

October 3, 1915.

My fund is like the widow's cruse - it never gives out. Somebody is always sending me something. I do hope they all realize how grateful I am and how much good I have been able to do. I have been very careful how I spent it.

A boy of twenty went off today. He had absolutely nothing warm to put on him, so I got him an outfit at Dunkirk. He was almost blown to pieces, poor boy, and he said that one sock was all that was left of his clothes. They provide them with necessary things at the hospital, but sometimes the supply gets a bit low and now it is so cold they need extra underclothing. When he was brought in they put him in a ward by himself because they thought he would not live through the night, he was so terribly wounded. His right arm was gone, he had a bullet in his liver - it is still there - and multiple wounds of head and body. But he made a wonderful recovery and went away very white and weak, but cheerful and confident that he will get something to do that will not require two hands. He has the Médaille Militaire and the Croix de Guerre, and his Lieutenant, Captain and General have all been to see him several times - they say he was a wonderful soldier.

Three of us went to Dunkirk by motor to get various supplies. We saw many interesting things on the way, and in Dunkirk saw the destruction caused by the bombardment. The whole side was out of the church and several houses were simply crushed like a pack of cards. Some of the nurses were in Dunkirk when it was bombarded, and they said the noise was the most terrifying part of it all.

The day we went to Dunkirk we saw a lot of armoured cars. Such curious looking things they are - some are painted with blotches of yellow and green and gray and red and brown so they cannot be distinguished from the landscape. We saw lots of English troops. I looked in vain for Canadians, but they are not far off.

It has been awfully cold so far and rains most of the time. We have decided that we shall just keep putting on clothes like the Italians do in winter and never take anything off.

We get wounded every day, sometimes not more than half a dozen, but as they are almost all seriously wounded we are kept busy.

There have been so many troops moving on lately, that we thought we would be left without anything to do. We have orders not to do anything that is not absolutely necessary as we may have to move also.

I believe the hospital at Divonne has been taken over by the nuns. I miss the lovely flowers that I had there. I share a small room with two other nurses and there is not much room to spare. We have boxes put up on end for tables and washstands, and there is only one chair. Some of the nurses have tents, two in each. We have had a terrible busy week. All the new ones that came into my ward lived only thirty-six or forty-eight hours - they were too far gone to save. Five went away cured, and they really were cases to be proud of.

I think it was the sweetest thing of little Mary Murray to send me her birthday money for my soldiers. I have been getting them fruit and cigarettes for Sunday. That is the thing that overwhelms me at times - the awful suffering every way one turns.

Last night I could not sleep for the noise of the guns; they must have been bombarding some place near at hand, for the whole earth seemed to shake.

The boys who drive the American ambulance and bring our patients in say this place is a sort of heaven to them they are always glad to get here. Mrs. T does everything she can for them. They are a nice lot of boys and are doing good work.

Some of the poor men who have lost large pieces of their intestines find the hospital diet a little hard.

Mobile No. 1, November 7, 1915.

Letter writing is done under difficulties here. I have gone to bed in order to keep warm and have a small lantern with a candle in to light the paper.

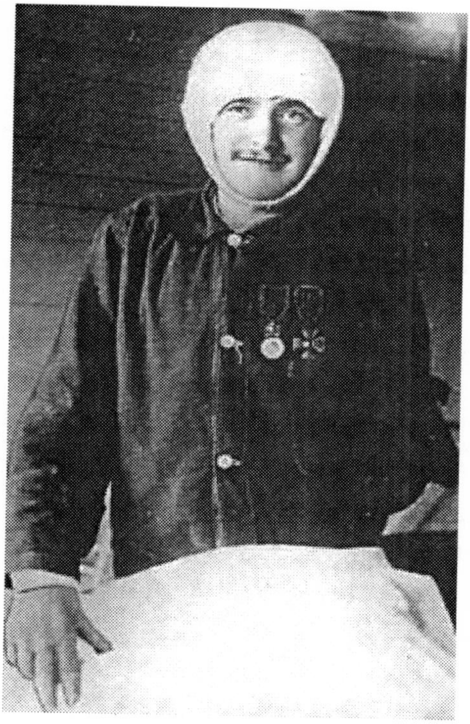

Thought to be a hopeless case, but everyone must have their chance, three doctors operated at once, amputating leg, an arm and trepanning. Now as happy as the day is long.

November 15, 1915.

I did not get any further with my letter for the kitty insisted upon playing with the candle and I was afraid we would have a fire, and since then I have been so busy I have not had a minute. We have had three glorious days and have appreciated them, I can tell you. It has been so cold and wet we have all been water-logged.

As for me, I have no word to express my gratitude for all the friends have sent to me. I am quite overwhelmed with all the gifts of money and supplies, but I shall make good use of them and nothing shall be wasted.

The wool which Mrs. S. sent turned up yesterday and I have already given half of it to the women in one of the villages here to knit into socks.

There is a dear old English colonel who has a soup kitchen near the firing line, and he is always looking for socks. He does a great deal of good, for he gets the men when they are carried in from the trenches and gives them hot drinks and hot water bottles, and warm socks when he has them. So many of the men have just straw in their boots and are almost frozen. It makes such a difference if they can get warmed up quickly. Poor souls, they have had a hard time since the heavy rains began. They are brought in here just caked with mud from head to foot.

Oh, how glad I was to get the cheque from the 'Red Cross' Society and the cheque from Miss C. I have written to her and would like to write long letters to every one who is so kind, but there is not time.

This Ambulance was established by an American lady who then gave it to the French government. The expenses of running it are paid by them, but I think Mrs. S pays the nurses and also helps out in the way of extra supplies.

On All Saints Day we went to the little cemetery and decorated the graves of the soldiers who have died in the hospital. There was a special mass and service in the churchyard and the General sent us an invitation. It was pouring rain but I would not have missed it for anything, and I only wish the mothers, wives and sisters could know how beautiful it all was and how tenderly cared for are the last resting-places of their dear ones.

It was a picture I shall never forget. The corner of the little churchyard with the forty new graves so close together, each marked with a small wooden cross and heaped high with flowers - the General standing with a group of officers and soldiers all with bared heads - the nurses and one or two of the doctors from the hospital behind them, and then the village people and refugees - hundreds of them, it seemed to me - and the priest giving his lesson - and all the time the rain coming down in torrents and nobody paying any attention to it. There were no dry eyes and when the General came and shook hands with us afterwards, he could not speak. He is a splendid man, very handsome and a patriot to the backbone - one of the finest types of Frenchmen.

Do not worry about me for I am very well and so glad to be here in spite of the cold and discomforts. Mrs. S's socks and bandages have just come.

November 28, 1915.

It is bitterly cold here, and we feel it more because it is so damp. I can't tell you how thankful I am to be able to get socks and warm things for the men. We can send things to the first dressing station by the ambulances, and from there they go to the trenches at once. Mrs. D's socks came yesterday, and I sent them off to Colonel Noble, who has the soup kitchen at the front. All Mrs. S's have been given away. It was such a good idea to have them white, for they put them on under the others and it often saves the men from being infected by the dye of the stockings.

This morning when I got up my room was like a skating pond, for the moisture had frozen on the floor and the water in the pitcher was solid. The getting up in the morning is the hardest, but after we get started we do not mind the cold.

The patients have plenty of blankets and hot water bottles, so they do not suffer.

Two Zeppelins went over our head yesterday, but fortunately we are too unimportant to be noticed. I suppose that is one of the reasons they will not let us say where we are, for there are so many spies everywhere that can send information.

An English nurse came yesterday; she has had most interesting experiences. She was in Brussels when it was taken by the Germans and was obliged to take care of German soldiers and officers for some time. She said the officers, as a rule, were brutes, but some of the men were very nice and grateful.

For three days and nights the guns have thundered without ceasing. I wonder what it all means?

My kitty keeps all the seventeen dogs that loaf around here in order. Yesterday she chased a big yellow dog, half St. Bernard, down the main sidewalk of the Ambulance. It was a very funny sight, for she was like a little round ball of fury and the poor dog was frightened to death.

December 5, 1915.

Last night we had the most awful wind storm. I thought our little hut would be carried over into the German lines. It rained in torrents and the roof leaked, and I could not get my bed away from the drips, so I put up my umbrella and the kitty and I had quite a comfortable night.

Ben Ali, the poor Arab who was so desperately wounded, was up today for the first time.

I have ordered six dozen pair of socks from Paris. My nice old English Colonel Noble (with the soup kitchen) is always clamoring for them. I think he saves lots of the men from having frozen feet. Madge S's wool is being made into socks by the women of the village.

December 26, 1915.

Christmas is over, and in spite of the under - current of sadness and the suffering the men had a very happy day. In my ward all but one were well enough to enjoy the tree, and they were like a lot of children with their stockings. Christmas Eve one of the orderlies who was on guard helped me decorate the ward and trim the tree, then we hung up their stockings. They had oranges, sweets and cigarettes and some small toys and puzzles and various things of that kind to amuse them.

I had a package for each one in the morning, and, thanks to my good friends at home, was able to give them some nice things. I had a pair of warm socks and gloves for each one, a writing pad and envelopes, pen, pencil, small comb in a case, tooth brush, tooth powder, piece of soap, wash cloth and a small alcohol lamp with solidified alcohol - a thing made especially for the trenches and which delighted them very much - also a small box of sweets, and to several of the very poor ones I gave a small purse with five francs in it. One poor boy said he had never had such a Christmas in his life; he is one of a family of seven, and says that in times of peace it was all they could do to get enough to eat.

Christmas day at four o'clock the tree was lighted, and one of the many priests who act as infirmiers here came round to the different wards and sang carols. He has a very beautiful voice and was much appreciated by the soldiers. Mrs. Turner then came in, followed by an orderly with a huge hamper containing a present for each man. They had a wonderful dinner, soup, raw oysters, (which came from Dunkirk by motor), plum pudding, etc. I could only give my men a bite of pudding to taste it, but they were able to eat the oysters and other things in moderation.

In the other wards, where there were only arms and legs and heads to consider, they had a royal feast. She also gave a grand dinner to all the infirmiers and men on the place - had a tree for them and a present for each one. We also had a good dinner and a present for each. She certainly went to a great deal of trouble and made many people happy.

The next day we divided the things on the trees and each man made a package to send home to his children. They were even more delighted to be able to do this than with their own things.

One poor man in my ward was so ill that I was afraid he would die, so I moved his bed to the end of the ward and put screens around it so that he would not be disturbed and that the others would not be disheartened by seeing him. He was so much better Christmas night that we had great hopes of saving him, but today he died. He was wounded in seven places and one hip was gone. The General came at four o'clock and decorated him. He roused up and saluted and seemed so pleased. In the evening the doctor came to do his dressing and he seemed much better. After the doctor had gone he turned to me and said, 'that Major knows what he is about, he is a corker.'

Ben Ali, my prize Arab, had a wonderful day. He ate too much and had to stay in bed today, but he has been wrapping and unwrapping his presents and having a fine time. He is just like a child, he is so pleased. He has taken a great fancy to me and asked me to visit him after the war is over.

We had midnight mass on Christmas Eve for the infirmiers and personnel of the hospital. One of the empty wards was fitted up as a chapel and a Franciscan monk from Montreal officiated. He is on duty here in the lingerie, and is a splendid man. He is delicate, has some serious heart trouble, so that he need not stay, but he came over to do what he could for his country and his services are invaluable here. His mother was in the north of the country taken by the Germans and he has not been able to get any news of her for more than a year.

We have had orders from headquarters to close all the shutters as soon as the lights are lit, so we feel as if we were shut up in packing cases.

There were a great many aeroplanes flying about today, so I suppose they are expecting an attack of some kind. It is blowing a gale tonight and I feel as if our little shanty would blow over.

It is hard to believe that we are beginning another year. If only it will bring a lasting peace! The boxes have not turned up yet, but they doubtless will one of these days, and we will be all the more glad to see them because we have used up everything else.

I expected to go on night duty immediately after Christmas, but we had such sick people in my ward they did not want to make a change just then.

It is blowing a gale again tonight, and raining in torrents; it seems as if it would never stop raining. The roof of one of the wards was loosened the other night the wind was so strong, so the patients had to be all moved out while it was being mended. Our barracks had to be propped up also, all one side was loose and the rain came in sheets. I frequently go to bed with an umbrella

January 16, 1916.

We have had orders to evacuate all the men who are able to travel, so we got rid of a great many - eighteen went on Tuesday, twenty on Friday and nineteen more are to go next Tuesday.

The roof nearly blew off my ward last night, so my patients had to be moved into the next ward till it is mended. I am going to take advantage of it and have a thorough house cleaning.

Le Roux, the boy who has been here so long and who has been so terribly ill, died on Tuesday. I had great hopes of him up till the last day. Half an hour after he died the General came to decorate him. I hope they will send the medals to his people, it seems hard that they should have been just too late to give them to him. The next day I went to his funeral - the first soldier's funeral I have seen. I was impressed with the dignity and simplicity of it. The plain deal coffin was covered with a black pall, which had a white cross at the head, the French flag covered the foot and a bunch of purple violets, tied with red, white and blue ribbon, lay between. It was carried in one of the covered military carts.

At three o'clock the little procession started for the cemetery. First came the priest in soldier's uniform, carrying a small wooden cross, on which was written Le Roux's name and the name of his regiment. One of this kind is always put at the head of each grave. Then came three soldiers with guns on their shoulders, then the car bearing the coffin, and on each side three soldiers with arms reversed; directly behind were two infirmiers and three soldiers with guns on their shoulders, we two nurses in our uniforms, then two officers and some more soldiers.

As we went down the road to the little church in R - we passed long lines of soldiers going somewhere, and everyone saluted. A few stray people followed us into the church and afterwards to the graveyard, where we left Le Roux with his comrades who had gone before. I had not been there since All Saints Day and it was sad to see how many more graves had been added to the line. The ward seems very empty without Le Roux, but I am glad that the poor boy is at rest for he has suffered so long. I am beginning to think that death is the only good thing that can come to many of us.

January 25, 1916.

We have been awfully busy, wounded arriving every night, sometimes nine and sometimes ten, etc. Tonight we have had only six so far, but will probably have some more before eight a.m., they have all been very bad cases. There has been a terrific bombardment every night we have been on duty.

My little tent nearly blew away in the big wind storm, so I had to sleep in the barracks - or rather try to sleep. I did not succeed very well, so today I moved back to the tent. From my bed in the tent I can see the troops passing on the road and aeroplanes in the sky. Today we saw so many we knew it would mean trouble tonight.

The trenches were bombarded, and some of the poor men who were wounded had to lie in the mud and cold for over twelve hours before they could be moved, consequently they arrived here in a pretty bad shape.

One of the men had on a pair of Mrs. D's socks. I had sent them to Colonel Noble and he gave them to the men in the trenches. It has been clear and frosty for two nights, such a relief after all the rain. The hospital is full of very sick men. I am glad to be on night duty for a change.

January 30, 1916.

It has been so cold and damp today that I could not get warm even in bed. I like sleeping out in the little tent and as a rule sleep very well - have a cup of hot tea when they wake us at six o'clock. I wear two pair of socks, beside the rooms are not so frightfully damp since we got up the little stoves; they get dried out once a day, which is a great advantage.

I am sending you some snap shots of my little kitty. We call her 'Antoinette' after the aeroplane, for she makes a noise like the aeroplane when she sings.

When I have a chance I shall go back to Divonne for a rest - it is too far to go home - but there does not seem any chance of it at present. The English nurses who have been here six months will have to go first, and we are more than busy. There are two new nurses coming next week - Canadians, I think. It is very difficult to get nurses up here, there is so much red tape to go through.

You must not worry about me, for I am really very well. The cold and simple life is very healthy, even if it is not always comfortable. I seem to be as strong as an ox and the more I have to do the better I feel.

It is joyful to hear that I am to have some more money. St. John people certainly have been good. A box came today from Trinity, it had been opened. There is the ambulance, I must run.

February 6, 1916.

We are so busy here that we scarcely know where to turn. It is just a procession of wounded coming and going all the time, for we have to send them off as quickly as possible in order to make room for the new arrivals. Thirty-eight went off last Tuesday and fifteen on Friday, but the beds are filled up again. The last ones we have been getting are so badly wounded that I wonder who can be moved on Tuesday. We have had wild wind and rain for the last week, but today is cold and clear and for the `first time in weeks it is quiet - the cannonading has been incessant.

Two English aviators were brought in yesterday whose machine fell quite near here; fortunately they are not very badly hurt.

The box from the high school girls came today, and it was like having Christmas all over again - such a nice lot of things there were. I shall have a fine time distributing them.

Here comes the ambulance. One poor man died in the receiving ward and the other two went to the operating room at once. They both have symptoms of gas gangrene, and I am afraid one will lose an arm and the other a leg.

In spite of the cold and wet we keep extraordinarily well.

Four new nurses have come, much to our relief, for the work was getting rather beyond us. Two of them are Canadians from Toronto. They know ever so many people I know. They sailed from St. John at Christmas time and saw so many St. John friends of mine - they said everyone was so good to them. We do not get a minute during the night and some days have been up to lunch time.

February 22, 1916.

There have been two big attacks and we have had our hands full. Since Sunday the cannonading has gone on without ceasing. It seems to be all round us. At night we can see the flashes of the guns quite distinctly, in fact the sky is lit up most of the time. It is like the reflection of a great fire - it would be very beautiful if one could get away from the horror of what it all means.

The aeroplanes were almost as thick as the motors - one came down in a field near the hospital yesterday - the wings were riddled with bullets, but fortunately the aviator was not hurt. We often see Taubes, and Zeppelins have gone over us several times, though I could not recognize them, but the noise was unmistakable. The wounded are nearly all brought in at night so we have our hearts and hands full. The other night twenty-three came in at once so we had to call up the day people to help us; seventeen were operated upon and all are getting well but one.

From the twenty-third July, 1915, until the first January, 1916, seven hundred and fifty patients have been cared for here and sixty six have died. I have had over one hundred wounded come in at night this last month, and as they all come directly from the trenches you can imagine what it means.

Such a fine box came from Mrs. S and F containing bandages, socks, etc., all most welcome.

The ground is white with snow today but it will not stay long.

It is very difficult to get nurses here as a command of the French language is an essential.

The guns are still at it, so there will be much to do tonight.

March 6, 1916.

We have had snow several times this week and it is snowing again today. It is very pretty for a little while but soon melts, and the mud is worse than ever.

I feel that I can never be grateful enough to the people who have enabled me to do so much for these poor men. I am going to order some more pillows, they are things that we need very much. All the lung cases have to sit up in bed and need a great many pillows to make them comfortable. Strange to say we have not lost a lung case and we have had some pretty bad ones. There is one in now who was shot through the lung, and yesterday they took out a long sibber bullet from under his rib; he will be able to go home next week. When he came in he was in very bad condition and he could not speak for a week. The treatment is to sit them up in bed and give them morphine every day to keep them perfectly quiet, the hemorrhage gradually stops and they get well very quickly. We have had a number of deaths from that awful gas gangrene; there is not much hope when that attacks them.

The bombardments have been so terrible lately that those who are wounded in the morning cannot be taken out of the trenches until night, and then they are in a sad condition. One day last week, just as I was getting ready to go to bed, some people came out from the village to ask if we could help a poor girl who had been burned. Mrs. Turner and I went at once with all sorts of dressings and found her in a terrible state - her whole body burned - so of course there was no hope. She only lived three days. I went in the mornings to do her dressing and another nurse in the afternoon. She was burned by lighting a fire with oil.

Things are too heavy now for me to get my holiday.

March 19, 1916.

Only ten admissions. All the efforts are being directed against Verdun. The defence has been magnificent, and if only the ammunition holds out there will be no danger of the Germans getting through; but what a terrible waste of good material on both sides.

Mrs. Turner has been obliged to go to Paris and has left me in charge of the hospital. I hope nothing terrible will happen while she is away.

The snow is all gone and we are having rain again.

My kitty is getting very bad and spends all her nights out. She has grown to be just a common ordinary cat now, but she caught a rat the other day, so has become useful instead of ornamental.

March 20, 1916.

I am left in charge of the Ambulance for a time and am a bit nervous, having French, English, American, Canadian and Australian nurses under me.

We had quite an exciting time yesterday watching a German being chased by four French machines. They all disappeared in the clouds so we do not know what happened. Today I counted eleven aeroplanes in the air at once as well as three observation balloons. One aeroplane came so close over the barracks that we could wave to the pilot.

We had a lot of patients out of doors today, some on stretchers, others on chairs, and others had their beds carried out - they enjoyed it so much. We take advantage of all the good weather. It is pouring again tonight and the guns are booming in an ominous manner.

One day last week I went to Poperinghe with Mrs. C. We heard there were some Canadian troops there and I was hoping to find some friends, but the Canadians had been moved; however, we talked with some Tommies, gave them cigarettes and chocolate and had a very interesting time.

March 29, 1916.

Just a week ago a French general was brought in wounded in the leg while he was inspecting the Belgian trenches. We were rather overwhelmed at first, but I arranged a corner of one of the wards and he spent one day and night there while we fixed up an empty ward for him. The next day his wife arrived and she is camping quite contentedly in another corner of the ward.

She, poor woman, has suffered much from the war but is very brave. Her eldest son was killed, her second son is ill at Amiens, and this is the second time the general has been wounded. The first time he was in a hospital for three months. Her nephew, who is like a second son, has also been killed, and his wife, a young woman of twenty-two, taken prisoner by the Germans, and they have had no news of her since September, 1914.

The general's home was in the Aisne district and is, of course, in the hands of the Germans. There is nothing left of the house but the four walls; everything has been packed off to Germany, all the wood work and metal has been taken for the trenches.

The day the general was brought in, the King of the Belgians came to decorate him, and we were all so disappointed because we did not know about it and only one or two of us saw him. He came in a motor, accompanied only by one officer, and we did not know anything about it until he had gone.

We had another awful storm last night - wind and rain. Windows blew off and doors blew in, and one poor little night nurse was blown off the sidewalk and nearly lost in the mud.

One day last week I was surprised by a visit from two Canadian boys. They were doing some engineering work in this section and when they heard there were Canadians here they came over to see us. One was from Toronto, the other from Fort William. I gave them one of the Christmas cakes and some cigarettes. They went away very happy.

I was hoping to get news of some of our boys, but they did not know any of them personally but expected to see some of the men from the Twenty-sixth in a few days. I told them to tell any who could to come and see us. I have been hoping ever since their visit to see B or S or D walk in some day. It is awful to know that they are so near and not be able to see them.

April 8, 1916.

A cheque came today from the De Monts Chapter, I.O.D.E., which gave me great joy. It touches me to tears to think of the way the St. John people have helped me. I wish they could have a look in here and see how much more I have been able to do on account of the help they have sent me.

There is a soldier who helps here by the name of Baquet; his wife has just taken three orphan children, the oldest six years old, to look after, in addition to her own four, her mother and her mother-in-law. There are no men left to do the work on the farm, and poor Baquet did not know how they could get along. I gave him one hundred francs and told him it was from my friends in Canada. He did not want to take it at first, saying it was sent for the wounded, but I explained to him that it was sent to me to help the soldiers and the soldiers' families. He said it would mean so much to his wife, she works from four in the morning till dark. They are the sort of people who deserve help, and it is such a joy to be able to lighten their burdens a little.

We have only about eighty patients at present, but they keep us busy. The two men who came in last have been so terribly wounded. We have had a number of cases of gas gangrene. They are trying to cure them with a new sort of serum. Two of the men really seem to be getting better. Four cases were brought in yesterday. One poor man died at noon, and I was glad he did not live any longer; another they had to operate on in the afternoon and take his leg off. He was in very bad shape last night but this morning he surprised every one by asking for pen and paper to write to his mother, and says he feels fine.

Our wounded general left today. He could not say enough nice things about the hospital. He said he was so glad he had been brought here, not only on his own account, but he was so glad to see how wonderfully his men were taken care of. The guns have been going incessantly for the past two days, and we hear that the English have taken four trenches. I have also heard that some Canadians have come over lately and our B may be only four or five miles from me. I asked the general if it would be possible for me to find out; he said he would inquire and if B is anywhere in reach he would get me a pass to go and see him. I feel as if I would start out and walk to try and find him; but alas! one cannot get by the sentries without proper papers.

I hope my fur-lined cape has not gone to the bottom. I think I shall still need it in June, for after two wonderful sunshiny days we are again freezing. Sunday and Monday were like days in June and we moved the beds of the patients out in the grass and others were on stretchers. We had the phonograph going, served lemonade, biscuits, sweets and cigarettes. They had a wonderful time and all slept like tops the next night.

I think I shall have to find a new job when the war is over, for I don't think I shall ever do any more nursing.

I am trying to find a lot of straw hats like 'cows' breakfasts' and cheap parasols to protect their heads when they are taking sun baths.

The dressings are taken down and one thickness of gauze only left over the wound, and they are left in the sun from twenty minutes to two hours according to what they can stand.

April 11, 1916.

Yesterday we had quite an interesting time with air crafts. The machine came down so close, that we could see the pilot and his assistant who waved to us that they were going to throw something to us. A package landed, almost in the pond. It turned out to be a letter tied up in a handkerchief with some shot as weight. It was from the English boys who were patients here for a while; they told us they would pay us a visit some day. We could see the machine gun in front of the aeroplane quite distinctly. In the afternoon there was another excitement - a German machine chased by several French. It looked from below as if they had got him, but they all disappeared in the clouds and we did not know the result of the fight.

At nine o'clock there was a terrific explosion as if a bomb had dropped just outside the gate. We all rushed out and could hear the aeroplane distinctly, but could not see it; no damage was done near us. We have just heard that the bomb landed just outside the village doing no damage.

Thanks for the toilet articles, they are a wise selection. What we before considered necessities we now know are luxuries. We have just got off a motor full of convalescents going home on permission. I hope they will get a month, some of them have been in the trenches twenty months.

May 3, 1916.

I got a lot of linen hats and Chinese umbrellas to keep the sun off the patients when they are out of doors.

The two Canadian nurses are a joy to work with, for they have had splendid training and are the kind that will go till they drop. We have a wounded German prisoner who was brought in three days ago. The poor boy had to lose his right arm, and was at first terrified of every one. He expected to be ill - treated, but now that he sees he gets the same treatment as all the other patients he is happy and contented and very glad to be with us.

I thought if I ever saw a German in these regions I would be capable of killing him myself, but one cannot remember their nationality when they are wounded and suffering.

I am sending you a photo of the Queen of the Belgians, who visited us and was very nice; she spoke so highly of the Canadians and of the splendid work they had done.

Paris, May 24, 1916.

I left Dunkirk Thursday morning in time to escape the bombs, and stopped off at Etaples to look up some of our friends at the Canadian hospital. Dr. MacL had left for London but I saw M D, and M P

Etaples is a real city of hospitals now. I saw the St. John Ambulance and the Canadian unit; they are both most interesting, so well organized.

Captain T took me to the station in a motor, for which I was glad, as it is two miles, and the walk over in the sun was as much as I wanted. Arrived at Paris at five the next morning rather weary, had a hot bath, the first in a real tub for eight months, and when I went to bed that night I slept for nearly twenty-four hours.

Divonne-Les-Bains, May 30, 1916.

I did not go to the Grand Hotel for reasons of economy. This is a clean little place and I am quite comfortable but I miss the bathroom and the balcony.

There are no patients at the Ambulance here for the moment. All the fighting is in the north and at Verdun. Poor Verdun - it is terrible there, one hundred days and still no let up - I think there will be no men left in France before long and then the English will have to take their turn. When will it all end?

Divonne is as beautiful as ever, and so quiet and peaceful one would not realize that there was a war if it were not for the fathers and sons who will never come back, and the women who are struggling to make both ends meet.

I have had news of several of my old patients who were here. Daillet, who was paralyzed, is at Vichy and can walk two miles with crutches, two others have been killed and many of the others back in the trenches.

I have not been able to sleep, it is so quiet.

Mobile No. 1, France, June 20, 1916.

Today I went over to Poperinghe to look up Margaret H. She is in charge of the Canadian clearing hospital and is doing a wonderful work. They have been getting all the wounded from this last fight - receive one day, evacuate the next, and the third day clean up and get ready again. It is wonderfully organized; the trains come right up to the hospital and there is a nurse for each car, so the patients are well looked after. Margaret has been mentioned in despatches, I believe. I am so glad, for she certainly deserves it.

June 25, 1916.

I went over for Margaret H in the motor. She went with me to the cemetery near the hospital and I put some roses on the grave of one of our St. John boys. I wish his mother could see how well cared for it is. Margaret came back to tea with us.

Today I have been specializing a man who has developed tetanus. I would almost wish that he would die, for he has no hands, and has a great hole in his chest and back, but strange to say he wants to live, is so patient and so full of courage. When I have cases like this one I am always so grateful to the people who have helped me in my work. If they could see the comforts that can be given by a bottle of cologne or a dozen oranges they would be rewarded.

Our medicine chef was a prisoner in Germany for eleven months. The things that he tells us makes one's blood boil. One cannot imagine human beings as brutal as the Germans are. When they came into the town where he had his hospital, they shot all the wounded that were left and eight of his orderlies who stayed with him. He expected to be shot also, but they needed his services so took him prisoner.

July 16, 1916.

Another rainy day and as cold as the dickens, but we are glad to get through the summer without extreme heat or a pest of flies.

My tetanus case is really getting better.

Last week I went to a concert given at R for the soldiers who are resting. It was one of the nicest I have ever been at. I did not want to go, for I don't feel like any kind of gaiety, but Mrs. T insisted. There were only three ladies present, the rest of the salle was filled with soldiers just from the trenches. The concert was held in a stable.

Some English and Canadian officers, who are on construction work near here, have been coming to see us. One is Major H, who was on the Courtenay Bay work at St. John.

July 29, 1916.

We are nearly eaten up with the mosquitoes so I have been to Dunkirk to get some mosquito netting.

Mrs. T gave a grand concert to the men on the anniversary of the opening of this hospital. Denries, from the Opera Comique in Paris, and Madame Croiza, from the opera in Paris, sang. The Prince of Teck was here and in my ward, he was so nice to the patients. We had French, English and Belgian generals, colonels and officers of various kinds.

NO. 3 Canadian Casualty Station,
July 31, 1916.

I got twenty-four hours permission and came out here to spend the night with nursing Sister Margaret Hare, hoping to get some news of B. I have found out where he is and that he has been on rest and went back to the trenches today. They are usually on duty eight days and off eight, so Margaret is going to send him word when he next comes off to come here and I will come over and meet him.

I do hope we will be able to make connection. It is so hard to be so near and yet not be able to see him. If he is wounded he will have to pass through No. 10 Clearing Station, which is right next to this. I have left my name and address at the office, so if he should be brought in they will telephone to me and I can get over to him in half an hour.

The patients here are so well taken care of. They have had a light day. I helped her a little in the dressing room this morning, saw some of the men who had come in last night, saw three operations. There is a very clever English surgeon here and several McGill men. It is a scorching hot day.

My tetanus patient is quite cured, is beginning to walk about.

Mobile NO. 1, August 14, 1916.

We have had a strenuous and exciting week. It began with a visit from the King of the Belgians, who came to decorate three of my men who had fought in the trenches with conspicuous bravery. He visited all the wards and talked with the soldiers. Like all the royalty I have met so far, he is extraordinarily simple - wore no decorations or distinguishing marks of any kind. We were all presented to him in turn and shook hands with him.

The next day we got twenty gas cases and several badly wounded men - one Canadian from Ontario and two English boys, one was a policeman in London. I asked the Ontario man how he happened to get to our Ambulance, he said, 'he'd be blessed if he knew,' he was working on the lines which run right up to the trenches when the warning for gas was given. He started to put on his helmet and the next thing he knew he was in a 'Red Cross' ambulance on the way to the hospital. He is getting on splendidly but we lost four of the gas cases. It is the worst thing I have seen yet, much worse than the wounded, and the nursing is awfully hard, for they cannot be left a moment until they are out of danger.

August 28, 1916.

I have met our boy B at his rest camp not very far from here. It was a joy to find him looking so well, and big and brown.

September 9, 1916.

Rain, continuous rain. The guns have been roaring without any let-up for three days and nights, and our little barracks are nearly shaken to pieces. We have had several warnings of gas attacks, but fortunately nothing has happened. One of the orderlies kept his mask on all night and everyone was surprised that he was alive next morning, they are the most awful smelling things you can imagine.

We have never seen so many aeroplanes as during this past week. This morning we counted eighteen in a row.

Mrs. T is going to organize another hospital on the Somme and is going to keep this one as well. She certainly has done a splendid work. We are all hoping that the fighting will be over before Christmas.

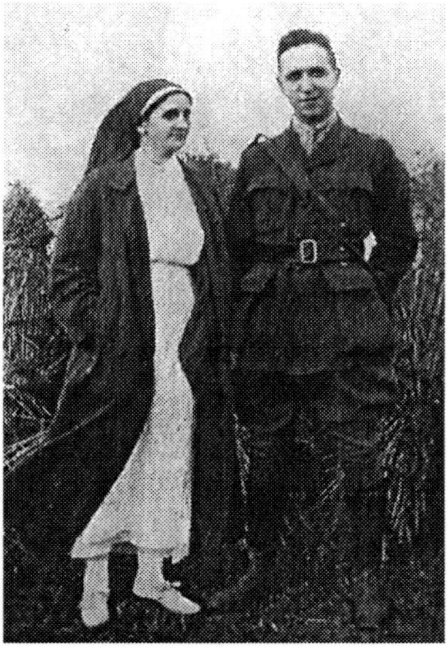

Nurse and nephew meeting in France,
One serving with the French, the other with the Canadian B.E.F.

October 1, 1916.

The rain has begun, so I suppose we may expect to be under water for the rest of the winter, but things are going well for us, so we must hope on; but oh, how dreadful it all is!

A stationary balloon that is not far from here, used as a Belgian observation post, was struck by a bomb from an aeroplane and we saw it fall in flames. The men who were in it jumped out with parachutes and both escaped without injury.

Broterl, the famous French sniper and poet, came the other day to sing for the soldiers. He is wonderful, and sang all sorts of songs that he had composed in the trenches. The men were enchanted, it does such a lot of good, for it makes them forget for a time.

One of our orderlies has just got word that one of his brothers has been killed at the Somme, another is dangerously wounded in the head, and a third has lost his leg - he has six brothers, all at the front.

One of the men in my ward got word of the death of his brother also. He was a stretcher bearer and was helping a German officer who was wounded. As soon as the German got to a place of safety he shot the poor man who had been helping him.

I am nearly frozen tonight and will have to go to bed.

October 9, 1916.

Our Bayard has come through the Courcelette fight safely, where the New Brunswickers did such wonders; but Oh, at such a terrible cost.

It has been very cold and rainy here. I am afraid the bad weather has set in.

Wish you would send me an aluminum hot water bottle for Christmas, another pair of Indian moccasins, and fill up the corners of the box with malted milk and maple sugar.

I shall never forget the poor little Breton who said when he saw me - as he roused a little when we were taking him from the ambulance, 'maintenant je suis sauvé' (Now I am saved).

I have just received a cheque from the Rothesay Red Cross. Since I began, my fund has never entirely given out, and I have been able to give such a lot of pleasure and comfort to the men.

If any one wants to know what to send me you might suggest Washington coffee like Lady T sent. It was a great success.

I am too cold to write any more, so goodnight. I wish I had some of Maggie's crullers and squash pie, but the French don't know anything about squash pies.

Our poor man with a broken back has been moved to a hospital near his home so his family can see him. We sent him on a mattress, fixed up with pillows and cushions so that he did not suffer at all on the journey. When I have any one who is so ill as he was I bless the good people at home who have made it possible for me to give them what they need. The guns are busy tonight, so I suppose we will be tomorrow.

November 12, 1916.

I have not had any home letters for three weeks. The Twenty-sixth have a great reputation here and St. John can be proud of them.

November 19, 1916.

We have been shaken almost to pieces with vibrations from the guns, these last three days. What must it be close at hand? On Wednesday we had a visit from the Taubes again. I could not sleep for the noise of the machines, so I went out to see what was happening. We could see the bombs dropping all around us, but fortunately none came very near.

November 26, 1916.

How we laughed over your stories. Send us some more when you have them, anything to make us laugh. It is strange how one can laugh in spite of everything. I don't think we could live through it if it were not for the funny and foolish things that happen.

I got a letter from our boy today. It is such a relief to see the dirty little envelopes with the address in pencil. There is never much news, but just to know that he is alive is enough.

December 9, 1916.

We have all been a little worried about Christmas this year, fearing that we should not be able to give the men a really good dinner. We have all been getting contributions and are turning them into the general fund, and now comes this fat cheque from the Canadian Red Cross at St. John for my beloved Poilus. How can I ever thank them enough for their generous gift!

All anxiety on the dinner score is now removed. We have about two hundred and fifty, counting infirmiers and men that work about the hospital - they are soldiers who have been in the trenches for nearly two years, or been disabled through wounds or sickness, or exchanged prisoners from Germany unfit for military service. They call the hospital 'le petit Paradis des blessés' and are so glad to be sent here. A man was brought in here the other day who was wounded for the second time, but he did not mind in the least about his wounds, he was so glad to get back. He is delighted because he will not be well enough to leave before Christmas.

We sent to England for some popcorn, and today the men have been like a lot of happy children stringing the corn for the tree. They had never seen it before and were much interested. We made quite a successful popper out of a fly screen and a piece of wire netting.

The other night we were talking over the various experiences we have had since the beginning of the war - the terrible things we have seen - the sad stories we have heard, and the strange but very true friendships we have formed - and we all agree that we could never have carried on our work in such a satisfactory way if it had not been for the gifts which have come from time to time from our home friends. The extra food that we have been able to give to the very sick men has made all the difference in the world to their recovery, and then the warm clothing when they go out, and the bit of money to help them over the hard place. You cannot imagine how much it means to them.

I remember so well one poor little man who had reached the limit of endurance, send when I found the sleepless nights were due to worry and not to pain, the whole pitiful little story came out. His wife was ill, his sister-in-law dead and there were six children to be looked after - the eldest a boy of eleven - and no money. As long as his wife had been able to run the farm they had been able to get along, but she had given out. The French soldier only gets five cents a day, so he had nothing to send them.

He cried like a baby when I told him I could help him. We sent off a money order for one hundred francs the next day, and I wish you could have seen the change in that man. That little sum of money put things straight six months ago and now everything is going well. But he will never forget, and both he and his wife have a very warm feeling in their hearts for the good people across the sea who came to their rescue in a time of need. When I begin to talk of my beloved French it is hard to stop.

January 1, 1917.

The men had a wonderful Christmas day. They were like a happy lot of children. We decorated the wards with flags, holly, mistletoe, and paper flowers that the men made, and a tree in each ward. You cannot imagine how pretty they were. Each patient began the day with a sock that was hung to the foot of their bed by the night nurses. In each was an orange, a small bag of sweets, nuts and raisins, a handkerchief, pencil, tooth brush, pocket comb and a small toy that pleased them almost more than anything else, and which they at once passed on to their children. They had a fine dinner: jam, stewed rabbit, peas, plum pudding, fruit, nuts, raisins and sweets. The plum puddings were sent by the sister of one of the nurses.

In the afternoon the trees were lighted and we had the official visit of the medicine chef and all the staff. After the festivities were over we began preparing for the tree for the refugee children. We had thought that we would have enough left over to manage for fifty children, but the list grew to one hundred and twenty-five.

The mayor of the village let us have a large room in his house, as the first place we had chosen was too small. We had the tree on Sunday afternoon and three hundred and thirty-one children arrived. Fortunately we had some extra things so there was enough of something to go around. They had a lovely time, each one got a small toy, a biscuit, and most of them a small bag of sweets and an orange. The oranges and sweets gave out, but there was enough biscuits and toys, but there was nothing left.

We are all dead tired, for we worked like nailers for the past two weeks; but it was worth while, for we were able to make a great many people happy, and now we are sending off packages to the trenches - things that came too late for Christmas.

We expect to move this month. It will be an awful business breaking up here, for all the barracks have to be taken to pieces and moved with us. We have begun to take an inventory, and to pack up, but I do not know just where we will move to, the papers are not in order yet. It is hard to believe that another year of war has begun.

Postscript

Editor's Note from Diggory Press:
We thought that the following item that we came across in our research may be of interest to readers. It comes from the Saint John Globe Newspaper of New Brunswick, Canada, and is dated April 26, 1926.

The Late Miss Agnes Warner

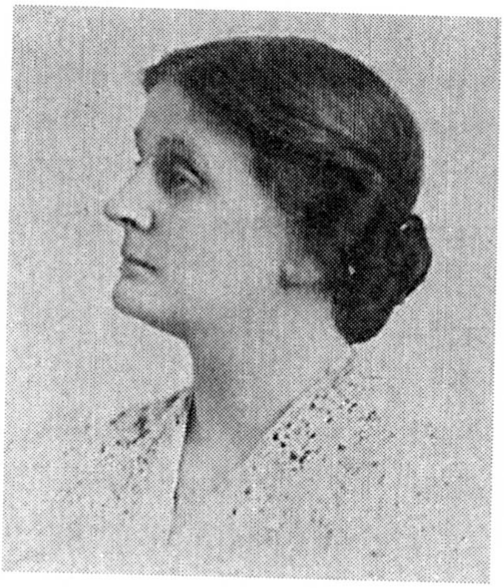

The quiet modesty of Nursing Sister, Agnes Warner, and the high ideal of duty, characteristic of a daughter of General Warner, and which were the constant influences in her whole life made it impossible for Miss Warner to speak of her own achievements during the years of the Great War.

In France when war was declared she gave her services and her knowledge to the little town of Divonne-Les-Bains, close to the Swiss border, and here helped in a way that has been but dimly realized by those who only know war from hearsay.

From the very outset of hostilities Miss Warner was attached to the French War Department, and she had received again and again assurances from France of the deep sense of gratitude that was felt for her untiring efforts on behalf of the soldiers and of the villagers with whom she was associated. Her interest did not confine itself wholly to the soldiers in hospitals for she knew the families of the wounded men, and many a poor French soldier went back to the trenches happier and more able to go on with the grim work of the war because of the money that Miss Warner sent to the poor mother struggling alone with the family, sustained by the indomitable courage and faith of France: many a word of cheer was sent by Miss Warner, herself overworked and worn, to waiting women telling of the husband of the son, the brother, the father from whom no word has gone for long months.

Everybody, said the author of *A Little Green Door* in France was better because of Agnes Warner, who was never discouraged, never unhappy, and who always in the empty depths of purse found the needed centime.

Miss Warner herself has told of the way she herded odds and ends to the amusement of her associates and how often she was able from the pile of apparently useless articles that filled one corner of her apt, to save the situation. For she was not then or ever in a large and well equipped hospital, nor on the highway of communication, but generally in Mobile Hospital No 1. at Bevereu so close to the French firing lines that the men came to her deep in the mud of the trenches and needing everything in the way of care and comfort. She had but one thought and that was of her men.

At no time had she said a great deal of the life she "endured." Her letters published in part in *My Beloved Poilus* are perhaps her greatest expression of these years in which she gave so unsparingly of herself. France was to her a country apart, the home of brave men and courageous women, a courage and bravery that could scarcely be put into words, but has enriched her life, just as she, all unconsciously has brought into theirs, the knowledge of a fine sweet, woman whose tenderness and sympathy, who knowledge and skill were freely given for them and their cause.

At the Sunday Morning service in Trinity Church, Rev. C. Gordon Lawrence made feeling reference to Miss Warner's death. He spoke of her as a woman of whom Saint John had to be proud. Her book, *My Beloved Poilus* Mr. Lawrence said, had been placed with the war records in the French archives and her service to the French soldiers would never be forgotten. Mr. Lawrence said that to her aged mother and the members of the bereaved family the deepest sympathy of the congregation was extended in their hour of sorrow.

On Sunday afternoon the funeral of Miss Warner took place. A short service was held at her mother's residence early in the afternoon conducted by Rev. C. Gordon Lawrence. The service in the church was at 3 o'clock and there was a very large congregation in attendance. The Red Cross Society was represented by a special delegation.

His Lordship Bishop Richardson read the lesson, and Mrs. (this is what is printed, but it likely should be Mr.) Lawrence conducted the service. The full choir of the church led in the singing of the hymns *Peace, Perfect, Peace* and *O Love That Will Not Let Me Go.* J.S. Ford was at the organ.

The pall-bearers were J. H. A. L. Fairweather, Percy L. Fairweather, Lieut. Colonel Alexander McMillan, S. A. M.

Skinner, F. M. Keator and Lieut. Colonel W. H. Harrison, MLA.

Internment was in Fernhill Cemetery and many beautiful flowers were placed on the field of honour plot.

OTHER BOOKS YOU MAY LIKE

A War Nurse's Diary:
Sketches from a Belgian Field Hospital
Agnes Warner, ISBN 1846853664

Mademoiselle Miss
Letters from an American Girl in a French Army Hospital at the Front
Anon, ISBN 1905363109

A VAD in France
Olive Dent, ISBN 1905363095

The Edith Cavell Nurse from Massachusetts
Alice Fitzgerald, E Lyman Cabot, ISBN 1846852021

Ambulance No 10:
A Driver's Letters from the French Front
Leslie Buswell, ISBN 1905363036

Observations of an Orderly at an English War Hospital
Ward Muir, ISBN 1846850355

The Angels of the Battlefields:
The Florence Nightingales of the U.S. Civil War
Brockett & Vaughan, ISBN 1846850428

The Nightingale Sisters,
The Making of a Nurse in 1800s America
Rosalind Franklin, ISBN 1846853710

The Nurse's Calling:
Practical Hints to Nurses in the Early 1900s
Harriet Camp Lounsbery, RN, ISBN 0951565591

The Edwardian Baby for Mothers & Nurses
Mrs. J Langston Hewer (Midwife), ISBN 1905363060

When The Nightingale Sang:
A Nurse's Life in the 1950s & 1960s
Rosalind Franklin, ISBN 1846853729

Only a Dog:
A Dog's Devotion to his Master in the First World War
Bertha Whitridge Smith, ISBN 1846853656

The Padre of Trench Street:
The Priest who gave his life for his men at Ypres
Alfred O'Rahilly, ISBN 190536315X

PLUS MANY MORE!

THESE TITLES CAN BE ORDERED FROM ANY GOOD BOOKSTORE OR BOOK WEBSITE

THEY CAN ALSO BE ORDERED FROM US DIRECT AT
WWW.DIGGORYPRESS.COM

A WAR NURSE'S DIARY
Sketches from a Belgian Field Hospital

Anon, ISBN 1846853664

The true account of a brave British woman's experiences while volunteering as a nurse with the Red Cross during World War One. Her diary describes in graphic detail the horrors of working on the Front in a war-torn Belgium.

Right in the firing line in the second battle at Ypres, she states, *'Our hospital soon became a shambles…our theatre a slaughter house. We started working that day, April 23rd, and we never stopped for about two weeks. Operations continued day and night with two tables occupied all the time...'*

However, despite the hardships, she still maintained her sense of humour and desired to see the beauty in things; rejoicing at finding primroses springing up amidst the ruins, and revelling in cantering on convalescent Blue Cross horses on the sand dunes in the bright spring sunshine.

One Christmas, she refused to let the Germans spoil her festivities. So, in spite of heavy shelling, she and the other nurses continued their game of hide-and-seek amongst the ambulance cars, the drivers running after them waving mistletoe.

THE CHILDREN OF FRANCE AND THE RED CROSS

June Richardson Lucas, ISBN 1905363192

In 1917, the Germans sent back into France through Switzerland all those they are unable to use in factory, trench, or agricultural work. The little town of Evian on the French/Swiss border received a thousand of such rapatriés a day. The Red Cross worked amongst these French or Belgian rapatriés, a large percentage of whom were young children. The American Red Cross focused many of their relief efforts on these children: many starving, sick and diseased, showing the effects of three years of dirt and riddled with lice and skin lesions.

June Richardson Lucas, a Red Cross Nurse, worked with her husband, Dr. William Palmer Lucas, Professor of Children's Diseases at the University of California, in the establishment of the American Red Cross work for the children of France. She spent much of her time at Evian.

"The children are so pathetic: many of them without their mothers, just sent along in a crowd in care of the older women, and some of them are too little to know their names and the old people have forgotten. To be four years old, to be six years old, and alone, 'Mother killed by bomb, father in the trenches'. Children come to us to get well and strong and 'wait for father.'

"Six hundred and eighty Belgian children arrived on the morning train, all these children, thin, sickly looking, alone; all of them aged between four and twelve. The boys were livelier than the girls – the little girls of ten and twelve, in charge of four or five brothers and sisters, cried bitterly. These children have been taken from their parents because their fathers would not work for the Germans and the mothers were willing to let the children go rather than see them starve. I have never seen anything more poignant than those little groups of children clinging to the oldest sister and brother as they marched down the little street. It was the saddest, the cruelest sight – little starving children, marching bravely along, singing, and crying.

"Men have been taken from 'No-Man's Land'– and it is a terrible place, that land between the enemies' trenches and our lines – but that little sobbing child comes from just as terrible a place, – 'No-Child's Land,' behind the enemies' trenches."

THE EDITH CAVELL NURSE FROM MASSACHUSETTS

The War Letters of Alice Fitzgerald, an American Nurse Serving in the British Expeditionary Force, Boulogne-The Somme 1916-1917

E Lyman Cabot, ISBN 1846852021

After the shocking execution of Nurse Edith Cavell by the Germans, American citizens asked the English director of military surgery to accept the services of the Edith Cavell Memorial Nurse from Massachusetts in the hope that it may be this nurse's high fortune to serve not only the Allies' wounded but their prisoners.

Funds were raised, and a nurse with exceptional qualities was searched for. One was soon found, and in early 1916, Miss Alice L. F. Fitzgerald was appointed by the Edith Cavell Memorial Committee to serve with the British Expeditionary force in France for the duration of the war.

From somewhere in France, Alice wrote: "I am in the thick of it, as this is the nearest Clearing Station to the Front. I am all but in the trenches! We are situated in a horseshoe, with the firing line on three sides. We can only walk a short distance in all directions for fear of getting shelled. The sky is alive with aeroplanes of all kinds, the scouts, the battle planes. . . some fly so low that they almost touch the poles of our tents. About a week ago, in the middle of the night, I woke up at the sound of the dropping of bombs nearer and nearer, until one came down so near that the vibration simply knocked me out of bed."

A VAD IN FRANCE

Olive Dent, ISBN 1905363095

In the summer of 1915, Olive Dent, a member of the St. John's Ambulance Brigade, left England with a party of one hundred other V.A.D.'s (Voluntary Aid Detachment nursing sisters)—for France. Olive describes her arrival at her destination thus:

"The car pulled up at the hospital to which two of us V.A.D.'s were allocated: a tent hospital situated on a racecourse three or four miles out of the town. We tumbled out to be received by the night superintendent nurse. We were taken to the night duty room, and in about three minutes time were wondering why on earth we volunteered for nursing service. It was 2.30 in the morning, the door of the duty room was swollen and would not close, an icy draught played along the floor, and the kettle refused to boil for some time, though finally some very weak tea was made. The sister lucidly and emphatically explained to us that she had no idea what 'people were thinking about' to send out such girls as we, girls who had not come from any 'training school,' girls who had 'not had any hospital training,'—what use could we possibly be?"

Olive and her companion were soon to prove their worth to this doubting superintendent as well as to the wounded soldiers that they nursed. Her story of her experiences of V.A.D. work and camp-life is while at times very amusing, deeply poignant.

"Camp-life in fine weather is glorious—glorious are the nights when the nightingale sings in the forest which borders our camp. Glorious are the times when we lie abed looking out on a moon-bathed sky with scurrying mysterious clouds, nights when we tell ourselves that there is no war. Glorious it is to sit and watch a rose sunset fade to mauve twilight, with a honey-coloured moon, —long drawn-out nights when one's life has time to pause, and one takes a moment to think. Then one loses the charm, turns sideways in the deck-chair, swallowing the lump in one's throat, a lump partly occasioned by the beauty of the evening, partly by one's sheer physical tiredness, and partly by the memory of a torn and gaping wound and of a magnificent young life dying behind a red screen in the ward yonder, quickly as the sunset..'

HARRIET WENT TO WAR

A Physical Therapy Nurse at French Front

Harriet MacDonald, ISBN 184685069X

As a young girl, Harriet MacDonald had been diagnosed with a crippling illness and given just six months to live. However, Harriet defied the doctors and, determined to 'make good', became a physical therapy nurse to help others suffering as she had.

In May 1918 Harriet sailed out on the "Manchuria" from New York to France with the first Orthopaedic Unit of twenty-four specially picked women. They went to assist the soldiers crippled by the war.

"Remember, girls, you will more supple a stump is the more use a man is going to have of his artificial limb, and it is up to you to let him have the most use of that limb."

"We were all ready to swear we would work our fingers to the bone for those maimed lads…." said Harriet.

Printed in the United Kingdom
by Lightning Source UK Ltd.
132738UK00002B/197/A

9 781846 853678